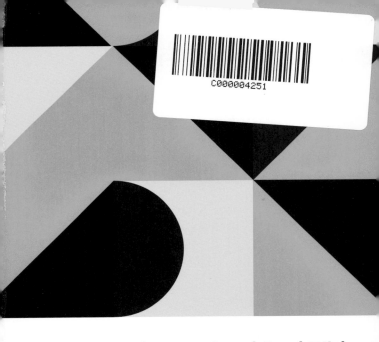

How to Understand and Deal With
Depression

 vie ———————————— **WENDY GREEN**

HOW TO UNDERSTAND AND DEAL WITH DEPRESSION

An Hachette UK Company
www.hachette.co.uk

Vie Books, an imprint of Summersdale Publishers Ltd
Part of Octopus Publishing Group Limited
Carmelite House
50 Victoria Embankment
LONDON
EC4Y 0DZ
UK

www.summersdale.com

Printed and bound in China

ISBN: 978-1-80007-426-2

Substantial discounts on bulk quantities of Summersdale books are available to corporations, professional associations and other organizations. For details contact general enquiries: telephone: +44 (0) 1243 771107 or email: enquiries@summersdale.com.

Disclaimer
The author and the publisher cannot accept responsibility for any misuse or misunderstanding of any information contained herein, or any loss, damage or injury, be it health, financial or otherwise, suffered by any individual or group acting upon or relying on information contained herein. None of the views or suggestions in this book are intended to replace medical opinion from a doctor who is familiar with your particular circumstances. If you have concerns about your health, please seek professional advice.

Contents

Introduction

It is normal to feel down now and again, but if you have depression, it can feel very different. You may feel low, find it hard to function, or even struggle to just get out of bed for weeks or months at a time. Around one in 25 people worldwide suffer from depression and it affects individuals of all ages and genders. But the good news is that with the right self-care, support and treatment most people with depression can make a full recovery – or at least learn how to manage their symptoms and enjoy a fulfilling life again. Depression isn't the same for everyone; the circumstances that led to your low mood, and therefore the way you deal with it, will be unique to you. The first part of this book aims to help you understand what depression is and to identify the possible causes of your distress. Part 2 offers a range of self-help approaches, as well as an overview of the medical and alternative therapies available, so you can choose the lifestyle changes and treatments that could work for you.

PART 1

Understanding Depression

This section gives you an overview of what depression is, its symptoms and its causes. People often say they're depressed when they're simply having a bad day or week. True depression lasts longer and, depending on the severity, it can severely disrupt your everyday life. Over the following pages you will learn about the different types of depression and their associated symptoms. You'll also discover the factors that may have contributed to your low mood, which can include excessive stress, insufficient sleep, poor diet and hormonal changes. This will help you to identify the likely reasons for your particular symptoms, so you can go on to find ways to deal with them.

What is depression?

Depression is the term used to describe when someone is suffering from a low mood, or has other symptoms like a loss of interest or pleasure in activities they usually enjoy. True depression causes feelings that interfere with your daily life and can come and go for weeks or months, rather than just days. The more your depression hampers your ability to function normally, the more seriously you should take it. As well as causing psychological symptoms, depression can have a negative impact on your physical health and how you interact with other people. Some people may only experience depression once in their lifetime, while others might suffer several episodes. It's true that some people view depression as a trivial condition that simply requires sufferers to "pull themselves together", but in reality if depression is left untreated it can become a serious health issue.

How depressed are you?

Depression can be mild, moderate or severe. Mild depression is very common and has some impact on your daily life, but usually resolves itself or improves by following self-help strategies such as those listed in the second part of this book. Moderate depression has a significant impact on your daily life. It might improve with self-help measures and you may need medical help with talking therapies or even antidepressants. Severe depression is much more debilitating; it makes everyday life challenging and can lead to suicidal thoughts. To recover you will almost certainly need both talking therapies and antidepressants. Your medical practitioner is likely to refer you to a mental health specialist.

Spot the signs

There are many psychological symptoms of depression to look out for and not everybody experiences all of them. You might feel pessimistic about the future and that there's nothing you can do to improve your situation. Your self-esteem and self-confidence might take a dip or you may find yourself becoming more anxious and tearful. Perhaps you've noticed you are more restless, irritable and intolerant of others, or maybe you are flying off the handle for no good reason. You might feel guilty about things you've done in the past or struggle to make even the simplest decision. For some people, just getting through each day and undertaking everyday tasks can feel overwhelming.

Physical symptoms

Depression can also take a toll on your physical health. Some sufferers lose their appetite and experience significant weight loss, while others turn to food for comfort and gain weight. Others might try to drown their sorrows with alcohol or use drugs to numb their feelings. Sleep disturbances are another key symptom, with some people having difficulty falling or staying asleep. Or you might sleep for longer and find it harder to get out of bed each morning. It's common to lack energy and some sufferers lose interest in their appearance, while others might find it difficult to complete domestic tasks or function at work. Panic attacks – which can be very frightening – are another physical symptom of mental distress. As well as anxiety and a feeling of impending doom, you might experience breathing difficulties, nausea and a racing heartbeat. Depression can even manifest as unusual aches and pains, stomach cramps and headaches.

Social symptoms

When you're in the grip of depression both your self-esteem and self-confidence can take a hit, and this can affect how you interact with other people. When you have a low opinion of yourself it's common to think that other people will, too, and you may start to withdraw from your friends and family as well as avoid social gatherings. However, the more you isolate yourself from other people, the more rejected and unloved you'll feel, which in turn can make you feel even more depressed. But you are not doomed to be trapped in this cycle of negative feelings forever – there are ways out. Part 2 of this book will support you in moving through your depression and getting out the other side.

Who gets depression?

Depression is a common mental health issue. The World Health Organization (WHO) estimates that almost four per cent of the global population suffer from the condition. This equates to around 300 million people.

Women are more than twice as likely as men to suffer from depression. This could partly be because women are more likely to see a medical practitioner and therefore be diagnosed. Plus, women are prone to hormonal fluctuations, which are often involved in low mood. Women also tend to face extra pressures from taking on most of the burden of childcare, perhaps while looking after an ailing parent and running a home, as well as holding down a job.

Men, on the other hand, respond to depression differently. They are much less likely to talk to family or friends about how they're feeling, or to seek help from a medical practitioner. This may be because men are generally brought up to put on a brave face and not admit when they're experiencing problems. Instead, men are more likely to bottle up their problems and use alcohol and drugs to help them cope. Drinking too much can make depression worse and raise the risk of impulsive behaviour, increasing the risk factor for suicide.

What causes depression?

Rather than having one particular cause, it's likely that depression is down to a combination of biological, social and psychological factors. These include a chemical imbalance in the brain, an inherited tendency toward depression, physical illness, the pressures of modern life, low self-esteem and a negative outlook. Depression can be triggered by stressful life events like bereavement, divorce, redundancy or serious illness. Money worries and loneliness – which many people experienced during the coronavirus pandemic – can also increase the risk of becoming depressed. Hormonal and physical changes during the menstrual cycle, after having a baby and when going through the menopause, can also lead to depression. Even changes in the seasons or low levels of natural light during darker winter months can help to create a persistent low mood.

Chemical imbalance

The theory that depression is due to a deficiency of one or both of the neurotransmitters serotonin and noradrenaline underpins the use of modern antidepressants, which are designed to increase their levels. Neurotransmitters are brain chemicals involved in the transmission of messages from one nerve cell to another. Serotonin is involved in the regulation of mood, appetite and sleep. Noradrenaline (also known as norepinephrine) is made from dopamine (another neurotransmitter) and is linked to mood and motivation. Levels of serotonin and noradrenaline can be affected by diet, stress and lack of sunlight, as well as low levels of oestrogen (estrogen) in women or testosterone in men. However, these chemicals can be boosted through many of the lifestyle changes suggested in Part 2 of this book.

Stress

Stress is what you feel when you experience pressures beyond the level you are able to cope with. One person may fare well in a situation that another might find stressful; it's all down to the individual's perception of it and their ability to deal with it. Many of us are leading increasingly stressful lives. Today's "have it all" society means living our lives at an ever-increasing pace, as we work longer hours to achieve a better lifestyle. The economic downturn caused by the coronavirus pandemic led to many people losing their jobs and experiencing financial worries. Bereavement and the breakdown of a relationship are also highly stressful life events. The body reacts to stress by producing stress hormones, which can alter the brain's chemistry and lead to depression.

Insomnia

Insomnia can be both a symptom and a cause of stress and depression. When you're stressed or depressed, you're likely to find it harder to drop off to sleep and more likely to wake during the night or very early in the morning. Lying awake and mulling over problems in the early hours only makes them seem worse than they really are. Lack of sleep stresses both the mind and body and, before you know it, you're in an endless loop of feeling increasingly stressed and depressed, and sleeping less soundly as time goes on.

Modern society

Social factors, such as living alone and poverty, play a part in depression. Single, divorced or separated people – especially lone parents – are more likely to suffer from depression fuelled by loneliness. While it doesn't affect all single parents or people living alone, the pressures of surviving on a low income and bringing up children on your own can often cause feelings of depression. Modern society is aspirational and materialistic. We're constantly bombarded with social media and advertising images of the so-called perfect life – successful, attractive people in designer clothes, driving top-of-the-range cars and living in big houses. For most of us, this kind of lifestyle isn't attainable and it leaves us feeling discontented, believing we must always strive for more rather than appreciating what we already have.

Loneliness

We humans are social creatures and a lack of contact with other people has been found to raise the risk of depression. This helps explain why many people found that their mental health suffered in the lockdowns imposed during the coronavirus pandemic. Having a partner or close friends to confide in is vital for good mental health, especially when you're going through a stressful time in your personal life or at work. When you have no one to turn to for emotional support you are more vulnerable to depression. People can feel lonely for all sorts of reasons, such as the breakdown of a relationship or the loss of a spouse. This is very common among the elderly, who often live alone and are housebound.

Loss

Psychologists also link depression with loss. Obvious examples are divorce, bereavement and redundancy. Less recognized forms of loss include moving to a new house, childbirth and getting married. While these are usually viewed as positive events, they also involve the loss of your old way of life. Loss is a part of life we all have to deal with – it's a process of letting go and moving on to a new phase. For example, it's normal to grieve after bereavement, as we come to terms with losing someone we care for, but if we bottle up our emotions or hold on to our feelings of loss instead of finding our way through them, depression can result.

Grief

Even though grief and depression share many of the same characteristics, such as sadness, loss of appetite, weight loss and insomnia, there are important differences between them. Grief is a natural reaction to loss, whereas depression often has no immediately obvious trigger. People who are grieving find their feelings of loss and sadness come and go, but they are still able to enjoy things and look forward to the future. However, people who are depressed experience a more persistent low mood, a lack of motivation or a lack of optimism for the future.

Internal anger

Another theory is that depression is anger turned inward. When life deals us a blow or someone treats us badly, some of us hang on to our rage instead of acknowledging it and expressing it in an appropriate, assertive or non-aggressive way. This could be because we're frightened to upset the other person, or because we think they'll be angry with us if we express our anger with them or the situation. Repressing your anger can leave you feeling low and drained of energy, as well as suffering from symptoms like chronic pain, which you might notice as a persistent backache or headaches, for example.

Genes

Research suggests that a tendency to suffer from depression may be inherited, and the genes involved in the way our bodies use the mood hormone serotonin have been implicated. Personality traits linked to depression, such as low self-esteem or being too self-critical, can also run in families. Genetics can play a part in conditions such as bipolar disorder, too. However, the science of epigenetics suggests that an inherited tendency toward developing a certain condition, such as depression, can be overridden by lifestyle choices including diet and the way we think, so your family history shouldn't be used as a reason for accepting depression as an inevitable and irreversible outcome. It's also possible that people copy the behaviour of other family members. Shared lifestyles – for example, the type of food a family eats and how active they are – may also play a part.

Bipolar affective disorder

One in 100 people suffer from bipolar disorder (previously known as manic depression), which is characterized by extreme highs and lows, ranging from great elation to utter despair. During a high phase the sufferer talks a lot, is full of energy and plans and has little need for sleep. During a low period the sufferer may lose touch with reality and experience delusions and hallucinations. Most people who develop this type of depression first experience it in their late teens to early twenties. A combination of genetic, environmental and physical factors may be the cause.

Hormonal changes

Many women experience a dip in their mood, known as premenstrual syndrome (PMS), five to ten days before their period. It's thought that cyclical changes in the female hormones, progesterone and oestrogen (estrogen) affect levels of the happy hormone, serotonin. Symptoms of PMS include abdominal bloating, breast tenderness, headache, anxiety, irritability and tearfulness, which end soon after menstruation starts. A more severe form, known as premenstrual dysphoric disorder (PMDD), causes more serious depression, irritability and tension and usually requires medical treatment. Dramatic hormonal changes during and after pregnancy (see page 26) can also trigger depression. Another flashpoint is the menopause, when levels of progesterone and oestrogen (estrogen) drop dramatically. Monthly periods will eventually end and this may trigger bouts of low mood, which can be balanced out with Hormone Replacement Therapy (HRT).

Giving birth

Some women are particularly vulnerable to depression after giving birth. The hormonal and physical changes, as well as the added responsibility of a new life, can lead to postnatal illness (PNI) – previously called postnatal depression. This type of depression affects around one in seven women after giving birth. PNI triggers much more severe depressive symptoms than the "baby blues", – a common but short-lived spell of unhappiness usually experienced three or four days after giving birth. PNI typically starts within two months of having a baby and tends to develop slowly. Often the sufferer doesn't realize they have the condition, which can make it hard to diagnose. Like ordinary depression there are often several triggers, including previous episodes of depression, hormonal imbalance, lack of sleep and a lack of social support.

Men get PNI, too

Men can also suffer with postnatal illness and up to one in ten partners experience depression in the first year of being a parent. It's thought the additional financial and emotional pressures of having children, as well as a lack of sleep, are to blame. Also, it's thought that depression can be "catching", so if one parent develops depression the other is more likely to.

A change in the seasons

Another type of depression – Seasonal Affective Disorder (SAD) – can develop in the darker winter months. As well as feeling down and more tired than usual, sufferers feel hungrier and crave sweet, starchy foods, which can lead to weight gain. Depending on the climate where you live, around one in 50 people experience SAD, whereas one in eight people can suffer from a milder form known as "winter blues". A lack of sunlight on the skin means the body makes less vitamin D, which is needed to produce serotonin, our happy hormone. Meanwhile the longer, darker nights encourage the body to make more melatonin, the hormone that makes us feel sleepy.

Eating habits

A balanced diet is fundamental not only to your physical health, but also your mental wellbeing. Your brain needs a wide range of nutrients, including fats, complex carbohydrates, proteins, vitamins and minerals to keep you feeling happy, optimistic and motivated, as well as improve your ability to deal with the stresses and strains of modern life. However, depression can affect your appetite and some sufferers lose interest in eating, which causes unintended weight loss and a lack of vital nutrients. Others comfort eat – especially sweet and starchy foods – and feel less inclined to take exercise, so they gain excess weight. Being overweight can be a contributing factor to depression, as it is often associated with a lack of self-confidence and poor body image. This can lead to a vicious cycle of depression and overeating. So, if you are feeling low, one of the first things you should check is whether your eating habits could be involved.

Too much alcohol

Some people use alcohol to drown their sorrows when they feel depressed, because having a drink can make you feel more relaxed and confident. But alcohol is a depressant that affects the brain's chemistry and can make depression worse. Heavy drinking depletes B vitamins and other nutrients, too, making a low mood even more likely. Before long a depressed person can fall into a downward spiral of drinking to make themselves feel better, only to end up feeling worse and wanting to drink more and more. There is more information about alcohol and how to moderate your drinking in Part 2. If you are worried that you or someone you know has a problem with alcohol, seek help from a doctor or search online for a local support group.

Too much caffeine

Depending on how sensitive you are to caffeine, consuming too much coffee, tea, carbonated caffeine drinks or chocolate could contribute to low mood and anxiety. Caffeine can cause rapid rises and falls in blood sugar, which may in turn trigger mood swings. Plus, too much caffeine can cause insomnia so people who don't get enough sleep are at a higher risk of developing depression. On the other hand, drinking coffee in moderation has been found to lift the mood and possibly provide some protection *against* becoming depressed. A daily intake of up to four mugs of tea or ground coffee – depending on the size of the mug and strength of the brew – is considered safe for most adults. You'll find more information about caffeine in Part 2 of this book.

Not-so-good nicotine

Both smoking and stopping smoking have been linked to depression. Smokers feel happier and more relaxed when they have a cigarette because it stimulates the release of the feel-good hormone, dopamine; but once the effects wear off they're left feeling irritable and anxious until they next light up. In the long-term, smoking is thought to have a harmful effect on the brain and increases your risk of depression. It's also common for smokers to feel down when they first stop because nicotine withdrawal leads to reduced levels of dopamine. Also, some people use smoking as a psychological crutch to help them deal with stress, so when they give up they find themselves unable to cope and become depressed. But these difficult first few weeks of giving up are worth it for the long-term health benefits. For advice and help with quitting smoking, make an appointment with your doctor or find a local support group.

Prescription and street drugs

Some of the drugs used to treat physical illnesses like heart problems, migraine, epilepsy and high cholesterol can cause or worsen depression. If you think you're affected by this, speak to your medical practitioner as there may be an alternative medication you could take that doesn't cause this unwanted side effect. The use of illegal or street drugs such as cannabis, ecstasy, or cocaine is associated with depression. While some people with depression may self-medicate with street drugs to make themselves feel better, the comedown usually leaves them feeling worse. If you need help with coming off any of these substances see your doctor or join a local support group.

Lack of exercise

Another likely reason why more people are suffering from depression is our increasingly sedentary lifestyles. More people than ever before travel by car or public transport, rather than walk or cycle. Working in desk-bound jobs that involve sitting for most of the day, means many people today are far less active than previous generations. A lack of physical activity can affect mood by allowing stress hormones to accumulate in the body, causing insomnia, which in turn can lead to depression. Insufficient exercise can also have a negative impact on muscle strength and general fitness, making it harder to cope with the demands of everyday life. You'll find details of how to incorporate more physical activity into your daily life to improve your mood in Part 2.

Disconnection from nature

Some researchers think that humans have an inborn affinity with the natural world and that modern society's disconnection from nature is the root cause of stress and mental health problems. Experts point to people spending an increasing amount of time indoors watching television, gaming and doom-scrolling on social media. As a result of this, far less time is spent outdoors – to the detriment of both our mental and physical wellbeing.

Speak to your medical practitioner

If you've suffered from a persistent low mood for more than two weeks it's advisable to consult your medical practitioner – not just to receive a diagnosis and help, but to check whether a physical condition is responsible. For example, depression can be a symptom of an underactive or overactive thyroid, anaemia or an underactive pituitary gland. People suffering from illnesses like chronic pain, heart disease, cancer, diabetes, Parkinson's disease, coeliac disease and multiple sclerosis are up to three times more likely to suffer from depression than those who are healthy. This illustrates the link between mind and body, and reminds us that mental stress and depression can cause physical health problems – and vice versa. If your medical practitioner suspects a physical condition could be involved, they may carry out an examination along with blood or urine tests.

Be prepared

It will help with your diagnosis if you prepare for your appointment by keeping a record of your day-to-day mood and how it affects the quality of your everyday life, along with any physical symptoms like aches and pains or headaches. It's easy to forget something that might be important during the consultation so make any extra notes you feel might be relevant. It might also be useful to research information about the antidepressants your practitioner may want to prescribe. You'll find an overview of the types of antidepressants you may be offered and their possible side effects in Part 2 of this book. It will help you to make an informed decision about whether to take them or not.

During the consultation

Doctors often only have limited time to see each patient so get straight to the point. Remember to ask if your low mood could be linked to a physical illness or any medication you are taking. It's important to let your medical practitioner know if you're taking a vitamin, mineral or herbal supplement, as it could be implicated in your depression. If they want to prescribe an antidepressant but you're concerned about possible side effects and addiction, ask if you can try an alternative, such as Cognitive Behavioural Therapy (CBT), which encourages positive thinking. Always ask if and when you should have a follow-up appointment. When assessing whether or not you have depression and the level of severity, your practitioner will consider the number and types of symptoms you have, how long you've had them, and how much they affect your daily life and interactions with other people.

Life is a rollercoaster

It's important to recognize that ups and downs are a normal part of life. Some experts argue that normal mood changes have been medicalized, leading to people being diagnosed with depression when they are sometimes simply experiencing a human emotion such as sadness, loss, grief or despair that is a natural reaction to a situation. While it's important to remember that we can't always feel happy, true depression is a very real and debilitating condition. If you're in any doubt, speak to a medical professional and get some expert advice.

PART 2

How to Manage Depression

If you have read Part 1 of this book, you will have hopefully identified some of the stresses and lifestyle issues that may have contributed to your low mood. The next steps are to learn what you can do to help alleviate and manage your symptoms, along with the types of treatments that are available. This section offers a wide range of practical self-help strategies covering everything from stress-busting relaxation and positive-thinking techniques to mood-boosting foods and physical activities. It also provides an overview of the medical and alternative treatments and therapies that could help you feel better, including antidepressants, counselling and meditation.

Spot your stressors

For a couple of weeks, make a note of situations, times, places and people that make you feel stressed. Once you've established what these are, consider each one and ask yourself whether you can avoid any of them. For example, if you find driving to work during the rush hour stressful, maybe you could start or finish work a little earlier or later, or carshare with a colleague? If you can't avoid a situation, you might be able to make it feel less stressful by altering your attitude toward it or by taking practical steps to help you deal with it better. You can ease the effects of stress by practising relaxation techniques such as mindfulness or doing activities that help you to relax and unwind.

Find your now

When you're depressed it's common to dwell on the past or worry about what might happen in the future. Doing this can make you feel even more stressed and unhappy and takes your attention away from what you're doing now, which can negatively impact the way you handle your present situation. You'll find it's much easier to concentrate on the present moment if you only have to cope with one thing at a time. By focusing your attention, it will help you to deal with the tasks and challenges you're facing right now. Then, when problems arise, you can take appropriate action. When you channel your energies into what you can do to resolve an issue, it'll no longer seem insurmountable. Even taking the smallest step toward a solution can make you feel more in control, which in turn dials down your stress levels.

How to practise mindfulness

It's so easy to rush through everyday life without stopping to notice what is around you. When you live in the present moment life becomes richer, because instead of doing things on autopilot, all of your senses are focused on what you're doing. This is known as mindfulness and can be applied to every part of your life – from eating your lunch to going for a walk. Here's how: When you next step outside, really pay attention to the colours, shapes and textures of the plants and trees around you. Actively listen to the birdsong and inhale the different scents and aromas. By really appreciating your surroundings and not letting your mind worry about other things, you should feel more relaxed and better able to cope with any difficulties you are experiencing.

Everyday mindfulness

There are plenty of other ways you can practise mindfulness throughout your day. At mealtimes really focus on the sight, smell, flavours and textures of your food. To help with this, avoid watching TV, using technology or reading while you eat. Eating mindfully helps with weight management, too, because you're likely to recognize when you're full more quickly and therefore be less inclined to overeat. Whenever you're having a conversation, actively listen to what the other person is saying instead of letting your mind wander. When you take a bath or a shower listen to the gushing sounds of the water and feel its pressure and warmth on your body. Notice the scent of your shower gel or soap as you lather it up on your skin. By taking the time to observe the small things, you should find yourself feeling calmer and more focused in other areas of your life.

Indulge yourself

Do something self-indulgent every day. It could be a long soak in a warm, fragrant bath with a glass of wine and a good book, savouring a few squares of rich dark chocolate, listening to your favourite music, watching your favourite TV programme or doing a hobby you enjoy. Doing something you find pleasurable and relaxing will help to distract you from any domestic or work pressures and will help to lift your mood.

Practise self-acceptance

Are you a perfectionist who is never satisfied with your achievements and lifestyle? Feeling that who you are or what you have isn't good enough can lead to unrealistic expectations, discontent and unnecessary pressure. Psychologists and spiritual teachers believe you can only be truly happy when you stop trying to achieve impossibly high standards. There will always be people who are cleverer, more attractive, slimmer, wealthier or more successful than you, but there will never be another you! You have a unique combination of strengths, weaknesses, successes and failures that make you who you are. Try using positive statements called affirmations, that you can repeat to yourself every morning. Choose those that suit your particular issue. Examples include: "I accept and approve of myself as I am right now" and "I have everything I need to be happy".

Be true to yourself

Many of us spend our lives trying to be someone we're not; perhaps following a career we don't enjoy because it pays well or because it is expected of us. Life is too short to spend it doing things that don't reflect who you really are. Being true to yourself means living a life that is aligned with your values, so ask yourself what matters most to you. What do you want your life to look like? What are your passions? What are you good at? People who focus on the things that mean the most to them are more likely to reach their full potential, tend to be happier and more fulfilled, and are much less likely to get depressed.

Go for gratitude

It's human nature to take all that is good in our lives for granted, whether that's a loving partner, good health, a fulfilling job, supportive friends, a beautiful home, plenty of food – the list could go on. Often when we experience things on a daily basis we stop noticing and appreciating them and complain about what we lack instead, which can leave us feeling discontented and miserable. Unsurprisingly, it's been found that people who are thankful for the good things in their lives feel happier and more optimistic than those who lament over what they don't have. Constantly wanting more can make your stress levels soar, whereas adopting an attitude of gratitude brings peace of mind and true prosperity.

Choose experiences

If you're fixated on buying more and more material goods you could end up working longer hours to earn the money to pay for them – and become more stressed in the process. The more you buy, the more you want, so you will never be satisfied with what you have. Before making a purchase, try asking yourself if you really need it or if you'll use it regularly. You'll likely realize you've been spending more money than you need to. Cutting down on spending reduces your risk of becoming debt-ridden and falling prey to the pressures that money problems can cause. Instead, try choosing rewarding pastimes that don't cost much. This could be anything from learning a craft to taking part in a sport. Or how about going for a walk, which needn't cost anything at all. It doesn't matter what you choose, so long as you enjoy it and it helps you focus on *being* rather than *having*.

Slow down

Many of us lead increasingly hectic lives juggling work, relationships, family commitments and a busy social life. We cram as much as we can into each day, dashing from one activity to another with a constant sense of urgency. This never-ending feeling of pressure makes us impatient when we have to stop and wait; maybe in a queue, a traffic jam or when the bus or train is late. Next time you're stuck in a line or your transport is delayed, rather than giving in to anger, impatience or frustration, try keeping a lid on your stress levels with some of the mindfulness or deep-breathing techniques outlined in this section.

Prioritize what's important

If you're feeling overwhelmed by the demands of work, your home, your partner, your family and friends, it may be time to streamline your life. If you often feel under pressure and stressed because of a lack of time, try reassessing how you spend it. Keep a diary for a week or two to work out exactly where your time goes. Next prioritize the tasks and activities that you must do or really want to do. Lighten your load by delegating tasks to other people, then ditch the non-essential stuff that you don't have time for. Now you should find that you have more time for the things that matter most.

Manage your anger

Anger can be both a symptom and a cause of depression. When you're feeling low or stressed it's common to have a short fuse and overreact to trivial misfortunes or irritations that perhaps wouldn't normally bother you. Practising some of the stress-management techniques in this section will help you stay calmer and react in a more measured way. It's also thought that depression can sometimes stem from repressed anger. So, when you're upset or annoyed about something, try expressing the way you feel in an assertive but non-aggressive way.

Assert yourself

Do you avoid expressing emotions like anger or hurt? Maybe you try not to voice what you really think or to say no, for fear of upsetting or annoying other people. Perhaps it's time to try a different approach. Being assertive enables you to communicate your feelings calmly and diplomatically and do things because you want to, rather than to please others. Your choice of words is important. For example, use "I" rather than "you" when you disagree with someone. Saying "I disagree" is less antagonistic than telling someone "You're wrong". Stating "I feel angry when you..." rather than "You make me angry" shows you are taking responsibility for your own thoughts and feelings. It's also less critical of the other person. When refusing requests, explain why without apologizing. For instance, if you're turning down a dinner invitation you might say: "I don't want to go because I'm tired."

Stick to a sleep schedule

Insomnia is both a symptom and a cause of low mood and stress. Adopting good sleep habits could help you to break the cycle. Going to bed and getting up at roughly the same times each day helps programme your body clock to function properly, helping you to drop off more easily. While it's tempting to stay in bed longer to try and catch up on sleep after a restless night, it's not recommended as it can disrupt your sleep patterns and make it even harder to get to sleep at night.

Create a sleep sanctuary

Make your bedroom a sleep sanctuary – a place where you can shut out light and noise, relax and feel comfortable. Light encourages wakefulness, so use blackout blinds and curtains to keep your bedroom as dark as possible. If you live near a busy road or your partner snores, earplugs should help block at least some of the noise. Your body temperature falls naturally an hour or two before bedtime in readiness for sleep, so keep your bedroom fairly cool – around 16 degrees Centigrade (60 degrees Fahrenheit) – to help this process. Where possible choose cotton nightwear and bedding as this will absorb sweat and help keep you cooler, especially on warm summer evenings. The scents of lavender, chamomile and neroli essential oils are naturally relaxing, so keep some next to your bed so you can sprinkle a few drops on your pillow to help you drift off.

Select sleep-inducing foods

For your evening meal choose foods rich in tryptophan, an amino acid your body uses to make serotonin – which is converted at night into the sleep hormone, melatonin. Tryptophan-rich foods include chicken, turkey, bananas, dates, rice, oats, wholegrain breads, cereals and dairy foods. Dairy foods also contain calcium, which helps the body relax; this is why many people find that a warm milky drink before bed helps them drop off more easily. Ensure you're neither too hungry nor too full when you go to bed, as both can cause wakefulness. Drinking alcohol close to bedtime isn't recommended as, although it may help you drift off initially, it's a stimulant so it may disrupt your sleep later in the night. It's also a diuretic, so you're more likely to wake up because you need the toilet.

Bedtime wind-down

Try to develop an evening routine that allows you to completely relax. This could include watching TV but you should avoid programmes that could prey on your mind later when you're trying to go to sleep. Reading, knitting, doing a jigsaw puzzle or listening to music are also great ways to unwind. Our bodies are programmed to release the sleep hormone, melatonin, at night when daylight starts to fade. Artificial lighting can hamper this process, so make switching off or dimming bright lights part of your nightly routine.

Soak away stress

You could try a warm bath or shower as part of your bedtime routine. Your temperature will rise with the heat and then fall again, which signals to your body that it's time to drop off. The warmth of the water also melts away any mental or muscular tensions, especially if you add relaxing essential oils like lavender or chamomile.

Tech curfew

Avoid using your smartphone, tablet or computer in the hour before you turn in. The bright blue light that screens emit can overstimulate your brain and hamper the production of melatonin, the sleep hormone, leaving you tired but wired. However, if you find that using a device before bed helps you relax, there are ways of minimizing the risk to your sleep. Most smartphones and tablets now offer night mode settings which filter out the blue light on the screen at night; you can also opt for black and white mode. Choosing to turn off notifications while you're asleep will prevent any beeps or buzzes interrupting your slumber.

Sleepy head

Only head to bed when you feel sleepy or you could find yourself lying awake for hours. Giveaway signs that you're ready to turn in for the night include watery or itchy eyes, yawning, feeling drained of energy, aching muscles and struggling to keep your eyes open. Following a wind-down routine and going to bed at roughly the same time each night usually helps you to feel ready to hit the sack. If you don't feel drowsy at your usual bedtime, try doing something relaxing like listening to calming music or a meditation app to encourage the process.

Switch off your brain

There's nothing worse than falling into bed feeling exhausted only to find that your mind just won't switch off. If mulling over problems or thinking about a busy schedule the next day is keeping you awake, try clearing your head by jotting down your concerns or writing a to-do list before bed. If you wake up during the night and find yourself dwelling on your woes, remind yourself that problems always seem worse in the early hours and that you'll deal with things much better in the morning if you've had a good rest. If sleep still proves elusive try some breathing and muscle-relaxing techniques. You'll find more information on these exercises in the next few pages, so you'll soon be able to drift off effortlessly.

Take a deep breath

When you're stressed, your breathing tends to be shallow or you hold your breath without realizing. Slow, deep breathing reduces your heart rate, relaxes your muscles, relieves tension and triggers the release of the happy hormones, serotonin and dopamine. Being aware of your breathing also helps to take your mind off your problems and is a simple form of meditation. The next time you're feeling stressed or anxious, follow these steps: Close your eyes and pay attention to your breathing. As you inhale slowly and deeply through your nose, expand your stomach. Hold for a few seconds. Now draw your stomach in, exhaling slowly. Whenever your attention is distracted by a passing thought, simply return to focusing on your breathing.

Relax those muscles

Relaxing your muscles is another effective way to relieve stress and tension, because when your muscles are relaxed, your mind will be, too.

- Breathe in deeply. Clench your jaw and shut your eyes tightly, then relax and exhale.
- Inhale deeply. Lift and tighten your shoulders. Hold, then allow your shoulders to drop, releasing any tension as you breathe out.
- Take a deep breath. Clench your fists and tense your arm muscles. Hold for a few seconds. Release and exhale.
- Breathe in deeply. Tighten your buttocks and your legs, including your thighs and calves. Hold, then release, breathing out.
- Finally, inhale and clench your toes. Hold, then release and exhale.

Let go of learned helplessness

Some psychologists think that learned helplessness can contribute to depression. This is where you feel you have no control over the outcome of events in your life. In effect you believe that what happens to you is entirely down to outside factors beyond your control, rather than your own actions, which you can influence. People who think like this are less likely to believe they can make positive changes in their life or be successful. You can tackle learned helplessness by challenging your negative thought patterns. This in turn will make you feel more positive and confident, as well as feel more in control of your life and less prone to depression.

You feel how you think

Cognitive Behavioural Therapy (CBT) is a type of psychotherapy that targets your thoughts and behaviour. It's based on the belief that how you think affects how you feel, how you feel affects how you behave and how you behave affects how you think. The theory is that if you think pessimistically you're likely to feel depressed – and if you feel depressed, you'll probably respond to events in your life negatively. This will then come full circle to affect your thoughts again. CBT aims to help you recognize this and break the cycle of negative thoughts and behaviour by changing the way you think.

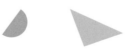

Turn a negative into a positive

When you're feeling depressed you're more likely to view events as all or nothing – good or bad – when in reality most fall somewhere in between. When something doesn't go the way you hoped, challenge any negative thoughts by recognizing they are just thoughts – your perception of events that you can control – not reality. Negative thinking is a bad habit that can be replaced with positive thinking. For example, you might view failing your driving test as a negative event, but by reframing it as a learning experience that will help you to achieve a pass in the future, you will be able to see it in a more positive light.

While it's not always easy to look on the bright side, it is possible to remain hopeful and positive even in the face of adversity. Remember even the most difficult situations can eventually have positive outcomes. How often do people say "It was the best thing that happened to me" a few months after being made redundant or having a relationship end? Now think back to a time when something bad happened to you, then try to think of at least one positive thing that eventually came about because of it. When you're facing a difficult situation in future, use this example as a reminder that almost every cloud has a silver lining. Adopting this kind of mindset can help you become more resilient and able to weather life's ups and downs.

Watch your self-talk

Self-talk is the continuous internal conversation you have with yourself. Your self-image – how you see yourself – is directly influenced by your self-talk. When you're depressed your self-talk is likely to be negative, resulting in a poor self-image, which in turn reinforces your low mood. If you have a negative self-image you will tend to brush off compliments, instead of accepting them. You'll be more likely to believe the negative judgements other people make about you – because they confirm your poor self-image – instead of recognizing they're just opinions and shrugging them off. To break the cycle and boost your mood, actively take control of your self-talk, making sure it's positive, so that you build a better self-image.

Be kind to yourself

If you constantly tell yourself that you're weak or can't cope with life, think of a difficult situation you've dealt with in the past, such as illness, redundancy, divorce or bereavement. Using this as evidence, you can now tell yourself that you're strong and you can deal with difficult life events. Next time you do badly at something and find yourself saying "I'm hopeless" or "I'm stupid", imagine what you would say to your best friend if they were in a similar situation. Perhaps you would tell them they tried their best or that they will do better next time. Now say that to yourself. With regular practice you should find it easier to treat yourself kindly and see yourself in a more positive light.

Act more, analyze less

When you're in the grip of depression, you'll probably find yourself overanalyzing your problems and questioning why you are feeling so low. But the more you dwell on your difficulties rather than confronting them, the worse they'll seem and the more depressed you'll feel. Instead, identify what you can do now to help resolve an issue. Even taking the tiniest steps toward a solution can make you feel happier and more in control of your situation.

One step at a time

When you have a problem, identify at least one step you can take toward resolving it now. For example, if you're feeling lonely think of ways you could make new friends – perhaps by joining a class doing something you enjoy, like art, cookery or yoga. Your first step might be to go online to find out what is available locally. If you have money worries think of ways you could improve your finances. Could you find a side hustle to earn more money? Could you manage your hard-earned cash better by creating a budget and sticking to it?

Take your mind off the problem

If you can't think of anything you can do about a problem right now, do something else that will distract you from it. Doing a few chores, going for a walk or calling a friend will make it harder for you to dwell on things. Who knows – perhaps a solution will occur to you when you are least expecting it.

Give yourself time to grieve

If you're dealing with divorce, bereavement or redundancy it's important that you give yourself time to grieve. Don't bottle up your feelings. Let yourself cry and express your anger or any other emotion you feel; these are normal reactions and part of the process of coming to terms with what has happened. Treat yourself kindly – indulge in your favourite foods and watch a TV show you enjoy. Perhaps booking in for a massage or going shopping for some new clothes will give you a much-needed boost. Eventually you will come through this and feel stronger. Then you'll be able to start planning and take steps toward a brighter future.

Reach out to others

Often when you're depressed the last thing you want to do is see other people. But meeting family and friends regularly is known to improve mental health, so it's worth making the effort. Talking to others can take your mind off your problems or even help you find solutions, whereas sitting at home gives you more time to ponder. So, reach out to other people; they may be able to share their experiences and offer tips to help you cope. If you want to expand your social circle consider joining a local group or class. There's bound to be something that interests you, whether it's singing in a choir, joining an exercise class or signing up for a walking group. Taking that first step may seem daunting, especially if you're feeling low and lacking self-confidence, but the benefits to your mental well-being could be huge.

Set daily goals

Setting goals can contribute to your happiness because this gives you a sense of purpose as you take steps toward them and provides a sense of achievement when you attain them. Whatever your long-term goals are, focus on what you can do each day to help you reach them. If you only focus on the end result, you might fall into the trap of thinking you can only be happy when you've achieved it. For example, if your goal is to get fitter, ask: "What can I do *today* to improve my fitness?" If your goal is to have a happy relationship, ask: "What can I do *today* to make my relationship happier?" By making your goals present-orientated you can engage with them every day and enjoy both the journey and the destination.

Find your why

Having a sense of purpose and meaning in your life has been shown to increase happiness and satisfaction. This could come from connecting with your spiritual self or a higher power, perhaps through prayer, meditation or maybe through nature. You don't have to follow a particular religion to have a sense of your own spirituality; spirituality involves finding peace and happiness within your unchanging inner self, rather than the ever-changing external world. This knowledge can give you strength and resilience during difficult times, as you realize that they will eventually pass. Having a sense of purpose and meaning could also come from having a particular role in life that you feel is important, such as being a parent or doing a job that you enjoy.

Food for thought

Most of us link what we eat with our physical health, but few consider the effect our diet has on our mental wellbeing. Research from around the world suggests that our diet affects the structure and function of our brain, which in turn influences our mood and behaviour.

Eating a Mediterranean diet – one that is rich in fruit, vegetables, fish, beans, nuts, wholegrain cereals and olive oil with a little red meat and dairy – has been shown to provide the nutrients your brain needs to work properly, and to reduce the risk of developing depression.

Healthy fats, healthy mind

Did you know that your brain is nearly 60 per cent fat? Research suggests diets that drastically limit all types of fat can cause depression; this means you need to eat enough for your brain to function well. One of the potential side-effects from taking statins to lower cholesterol – a type of fat found in certain foods and produced by the liver from other fats – is mood changes. Interestingly, cholesterol is used by the body to make vitamin D and we know that low levels of this vitamin are linked with depression. For good mental health it's important you include the right types of fat in your diet. Unhealthy saturated and trans (hydrogenated) fats, found in processed foods like pies, cakes and biscuits, should be avoided or eaten sparingly. However, polyunsaturated fats are vital for a healthy mind. Some fats can be made in the body from other substances, but polyunsaturated fats can't – you have to get them from food – so they're known as essential fats, or EFAs.

Up your omegas

There are two main types of EFAs (polyunsaturated fats) – omega-3 and omega-6. Omega-3s are found in oily fish and dark-green leafy vegetables, as well as nuts, seeds and some plant seed oils, such as flax and rapeseed. Plant seed oils, like sunflower and rapeseed, and meat also supply omega-6 fats. Your brain needs both types of EFA to function properly, but omega-3s are especially important for your mental wellbeing, as they are used in the body alongside vitamin D to make serotonin, the happy hormone.

Beat the sugar blues

Your brain needs a steady supply of glucose (sugar) to work efficiently. Processed foods like pastries, biscuits, sugary drinks and chocolate are broken down quickly, causing your blood sugar to rise rapidly – and to fall just as fast. This leaves you feeling hungry and craving more sugary foods, and the cycle repeats. Rapid rises and falls in your blood sugar can lead to mood swings. To get off this emotional rollercoaster keep refined foods to a minimum. Instead base your meals on wholegrains, proteins, fruit and vegetables, nuts, seeds and healthy fats. These foods take longer to break down, keeping your blood sugar steady and sugar cravings at bay. They also supply the vitamins and minerals you need for a happy disposition – and because they keep you feeling full for longer they help you to stay at a healthy weight, which also benefits your mental health.

Good mood foods

Eating protein-rich foods like eggs, fish, poultry, dairy foods, lean meats, nuts, seeds, beans and lentils, with unrefined carbohydrates such as wholegrain rice and granary bread, helps to fight depression in three ways. Firstly, these foods slow down the rate at which carbohydrates are broken down in the bloodstream, helping to maintain a steady blood sugar and balanced mood. Proteins also provide the amino acids tryptophan and phenylalanine. The brain uses these to make the happy hormone, serotonin, along with the motivating hormones, dopamine, noradrenaline and adrenaline, which we know are needed for mental wellbeing. Finally, carbohydrates help the brain to absorb tryptophan and phenylalanine from protein foods.

Eat a rainbow

Eating a variety of different coloured fruits and vegetables will ensure you get a wide range of antioxidants, including beta carotene (a type of vitamin A) and vitamins C and E. Antioxidants protect the cells in your brain and body against the damaging effects of pollutants. Fruit and vegetables also supply other nutrients such as the B vitamins and minerals your body needs to make neurotransmitters – the brain's chemical messengers. For example, the yellow and orange pigments in sweetcorn, cantaloupe melons, carrots, sweet potatoes, butternut squash and pumpkins supply beta carotene; while blue, purple and red-hued fruits such as blueberries, plums, cranberries, raspberries and strawberries provide another group of antioxidants called anthocyanins.

B vitamin boost

B vitamins are crucial for mental and emotional wellbeing, as the body uses them to make those all-important neurotransmitters: the happy hormone serotonin and get-up-and-go noradrenaline. As B vitamins are water-soluble, they can't be stored in the body, so you need to get them from the foods you eat each day. A balanced diet of meat, fish, eggs, dairy foods, wholegrains and vegetables – as well as citrus fruits, beans, peas, lentils, nuts and seeds – should supply enough B vitamins for most people's needs. But if you eat a lot of refined, processed foods, or you don't eat eggs or dairy foods, you may go short. Your need for these nutrients also shoots up if you're stressed or if you're a heavy drinker or smoker. In any of these scenarios, taking a vitamin B complex supplement may be beneficial.

Sunshine vitamin

We saw in Part 1 of the book how vitamin D deficiency may be involved in depression – especially Seasonal Affective Disorder (SAD) – because it's linked to low serotonin levels. This vitamin also helps the body to absorb calcium, which plays a part in mood, too. Exposing your skin to short daily spells of sunlight (without sun cream) is the best way to boost your vitamin D levels. Fresh or canned oily fish, as well as eggs, red meat and mushrooms, supply small amounts while margarines, bread, cereals and powdered milk are fortified with it. As many of us miss out on this vitamin – especially in the winter gloom – consider taking a supplement. Experts recommend a daily dose of 10 mcg for everyone over the age of one. Another option is light therapy, which involves exposure to a special light that mimics sunlight using a light box or a desk lamp, for example.

Mind your minerals

To feel happy and relaxed, you need both magnesium and calcium. Going short of either of these minerals can leave you feeling tense, anxious and miserable. Both magnesium and calcium are found in green leafy vegetables like spinach, broccoli and kale, as well as nuts, seeds and beans – including baked beans. You can even top up your magnesium levels by indulging in some dark chocolate. Wholegrain bread and cereals, bananas and avocados are great sources, too. But avoid drinking too much alcohol; having more than the recommended 14 units a week makes it harder for your body to absorb magnesium. Carbonated drinks are also bad news because they contain phosphates, which have the same effect. You can also soak up magnesium and ease tight muscles by adding one or two cups of Epsom salts to your bath. For calcium, dairy foods are a rich source – as are plant-based alternatives, which are fortified with it. Aim to drink milk and eat some cheese or yogurt every day. Other foods that supply calcium include canned fish – if you eat the bones – as well as bread in countries like the UK where flour is fortified with calcium. Calcium is also found in tap water, especially in hard water areas, and in some bottled waters. As well as vitamin D and magnesium, good bacteria (lactobacillus, bifidobacteria, acidophilus) found in bio yogurts and probiotic drinks, will also help your body to absorb this important mineral.

Mood-enhancing minerals

There are plenty of other minerals you can use to lift your mood, such as chromium, selenium, zinc and iron. Chromium, selenium and zinc boost serotonin and noradrenaline – the neurotransmitters we need for happiness. Chromium also balances mood by helping to keep the blood sugar steady, while selenium is thought to protect the nerve cells in the brain from inflammation. Zinc helps the body to deal with stress and iron is involved in carrying oxygen around the body – a lack of it has been linked to low mood. The best way to ensure you get enough of these important minerals is to eat a healthy, balanced diet that focuses on eggs, meat, seafood, nuts, seeds, wholegrains, fresh or dried fruit and vegetables.

Moderate your drinking

People suffering from depression or anxiety are twice as likely to drink heavily, probably in an attempt to make themselves feel better. But alcohol has a depressant effect, so it can leave you feeling even more miserable. Your sleep is likely to be disturbed by the urge to visit the bathroom, too, as alcohol is a diuretic. It's also a toxin that your liver deals with by using the B vitamin thiamine, zinc and other nutrients, leaving your reserves depleted; this can make you feel low and irritable and is especially harmful if you have a poor diet and are already short of these nutrients. The recommended weekly alcohol intake is 14 units, so try to stick to this. This equates to six pints of 4 per cent beer, six small glasses of 13.4 per cent wine, or seven double measures of 40 per cent spirits.

Curb the caffeine

Caffeine is a stimulant found in coffee, tea, cola and chocolate. In moderation it can lift your mood and make you feel more alert and motivated. However, heavy caffeine consumption can leave you jittery and anxious, so it's best to limit your intake to no more than 400 mg a day. This is equal to around four mugs of tea or ground coffee – depending on the size of the mug and strength of the brew. A can of cola contains roughly 40 mg of caffeine. Dark chocolate has up to 50 mg of caffeine per 50 g (2 oz), while the same amount of milk chocolate has roughly half that. Bear in mind, too, that if your body metabolizes caffeine slowly, you may have problems drifting off at night, which could also have a negative impact on your mental health. If you're affected, avoid drinking tea, coffee or cola, or eating chocolate after 2 p.m. Instead opt for decaffeinated tea and coffee or caffeine-free herbal teas. For a chocolate fix choose white chocolate, which is caffeine-free.

Stay hydrated

Your brain is around 80 per cent water, so even mild dehydration can affect your mental wellbeing. Psychological symptoms of dehydration to watch out for include depression, restlessness and irritability. Experts recommend 1.2 litres (2 pints) – or six to eight glasses – of fluid daily. This sounds like a lot, but you can get water from the food you eat, too. Fruits such as oranges, apples, blueberries and watermelons and vegetables like cucumbers, courgettes, iceberg lettuce, tomatoes and mushrooms supply at least one-fifth of your fluid requirements. Tea and coffee can be counted as part of your intake as they still contribute fluid, despite having a slightly diuretic effect. But because they also contain caffeine, it's best not to drink too many cups.

Herbal helpers

St John's Wort is a hedgerow plant with yellow flowers that has been used for centuries to improve mental wellbeing. It's thought the active ingredient, hypericin, keeps mood-enhancing serotonin and noradrenaline in the brain for longer by blocking an enzyme that destroys them. St John's Wort has been shown to be as effective as antidepressants for treating mild to moderate depression and with fewer side effects. However, if you're taking any kind of medication, seek advice from your medical practitioner or pharmacist before taking this supplement, as it can react with several commonly prescribed drugs, including the contraceptive pill, anti-epileptic drugs, warfarin and the antibiotic, tetracycline. It shouldn't be taken with antidepressants nor by anyone with bipolar disorder. A rare side effect is increased sensitivity to sunlight.

5-HTP is a supplement usually made from seeds from the Griffonia plant from West Africa. The body uses 5-HTP to make the happy hormone, serotonin, and it's been found to lift mood and promote sound sleep. Keep in mind that 5-HTP shouldn't be taken with other antidepressants, with weight loss drugs or if you're pregnant. If you suffer from anxiety you may experience a temporary worsening of symptoms before noticing an improvement.

Move to lift your mood

It's common to feel tired and sluggish when you're depressed but getting more active will help lift your mood. The World Health Organization (WHO) recognizes that being physically active can help to both prevent and ease depression and anxiety. Exercise uses up the fight or flight hormones, adrenaline and cortisol, that are released when you're feeling stressed. During physical activity your body produces the happy hormone, serotonin, along with endorphins – chemicals that act as natural antidepressants. Exercise boosts blood-flow to the brain, too, which improves your oxygen levels. And when you're exercising you're less likely to dwell on problems. People who take regular exercise tend to have higher self-esteem, possibly because they have a more positive body image. Joining an exercise class or a gym is also a great way to meet other people with similar interests to you, which can have a beneficial effect on your mental health. But you don't have to go to the gym to be more active, there are lots of other ways you can fit more exercise into your daily routine.

Housework-out

Doing the housework is an effective way of fitting physical activity into your daily routine and improving your mental well-being at the same time. Tidying, vacuuming, dusting and cleaning not only give the body a good workout but have also been shown to reduce the risk of suffering from depression and anxiety. It's thought the repetitive nature of cleaning can be calming, while seeing the results of your endeavours can be satisfying and gives you a sense of achievement, which dials up your self-esteem. Music also has the power to lift your mood, so try doing the chores to the sound of your favourite tunes. But if cleaning a whole room or home seems overwhelming, start small and choose a single drawer or tabletop to clear up.

Walk back to happiness

Walking can improve your mood and general fitness, and with a bit of thought you can easily fit it into your daily life – even if you're really busy. Why not get off the bus a few stops earlier and walk the rest of the way? Or leave the car at home for short distances and take the stairs whenever you can. At work, take a stroll on your lunch break and get up from your desk at every opportunity. Go and speak to colleagues instead of emailing them and maybe offer to make them a cup of tea. Head to the water dispenser for a refill every couple of hours as your brain will benefit from the extra hydration, too. These little bouts of exercise will soon mount up to make a real difference to your daily activity levels.

Go green

It's thought that we all have an innate affinity with nature and that our disconnection from it is one of the causes of mental health issues. Exercising outdoors in a green space engages all of the senses and anchors you in the present moment, helping to distract you from any problems. Being outside can also help to change your perspective by reminding you there's a big world out there. Getting outdoors brings the benefits of exposure to sunlight, such as higher levels of mood-boosting serotonin and vitamin D, along with sounder sleep, too. Being close to nature also exposes you to good bacteria found in soil, which is believed to lift your mood.

Gardening therapy

Gardening is a great way to get active and connect with nature as it requires you to focus on what you're doing rather than on your concerns. Cultivating plants and flowers is creative and can bring a sense of achievement, which is also good for your self-esteem. Don't worry if you don't have a garden, even tending a few potted plants and flowers in your backyard or growing some houseplants will bring similar benefits. You could even consider volunteering at a community garden. As well as providing a space to grow fruit, vegetables and plants, it brings the added advantage of meeting like-minded people.

On your bike

As well as being an efficient and environmentally friendly form of transport, cycling offers great mood-boosting benefits. It's also a fun way to take regular exercise and unwind while enjoying the great outdoors. Concentrating on the rhythmic, pedalling action can distract you from your troubles and put your mind into a meditative-like state. Many cyclists say that personal problems seem easier to resolve after they've been out for a ride. When you're feeling low it's often hard to feel motivated to exercise, so start with short trips and gradually build up to longer ones. If you feel able, you could join a cycling group to enjoy the social benefits of being on two wheels, too. There could be some scenic spaces near you just waiting to be explored, so why not get on your bike and cycle your way to a happier you?

Make a splash

Swimming is an all-round exercise that benefits both your physical and mental wellbeing. Focusing on each stroke and breath is a form of mindfulness that soothes away stress and anxiety and improves your mood and sleep patterns. The blue hue of the water is believed to relax the mind because the colour is found throughout the natural world and will remind you of both the sea and sky. This might explain why many people find being in or near water so therapeutic. Why not take the plunge and pop down to your local swimming pool? Consider signing up for a membership to get motivated to take a regular dip. If you can swim for just half an hour, one to three times a week, you'll soon notice the benefits. If you prefer to swim in the sea take care to choose a lifeguarded area and avoid going out of your depth.

Get in the flow with yoga

Aimed at improving posture, balance, strength and flexibility, yoga has also been found to brighten the mood and ease other symptoms of depression like insomnia, aches and pains and fatigue. Yoga involves performing asanas (poses) slowly and deliberately, while coordinating your movements with deep inhaling and exhaling. Holding each pose for a minute or two lengthens and strengthens your muscles and helps build endurance. A session usually ends with a guided meditation designed to clear your mind and invoke a sense of calm. Yoga can boost both your mental and physical wellbeing, making it a great form of mind-body exercise. A quick online search should help you find a local class, whatever your ability.

Mountain pose

The Mountain pose is especially good for improving your posture, which is believed to boost mood and self-esteem. The upward motion of the arms is also thought to lift the spirits. Stand tall with your feet hip distance apart, lift your body up through your legs and torso. Inhale then, keeping your arms parallel, stretch them as high as you can above your head. As you do so, lengthen and spread your fingers and toes. Exhale slowly, then keep breathing in and out slowly and rhythmically while holding the pose for one minute.

Pick Pilates

Pilates is a low-impact, mind-body exercise aimed at developing the core (abdominal) muscles, as well as lengthening and strengthening every muscle in the body. Practising Pilates regularly promotes good posture, which has an uplifting effect on mood and releases muscular tension. By encouraging deep controlled breathing, it also helps to relieve stress and anxiety and improve sleep quality. While Pilates has some similarities to yoga, it differs in that the exercises are carried out in a flowing movement and don't involve static poses or meditation. You are likely to find a Pilates teacher locally.

Try tai chi

Tai chi, often described as a moving meditation, is an ancient Chinese art believed to promote both mental and physical wellbeing. Each movement flows into the next and is executed in a slow and mindful way, while breathing deeply. There is evidence that regular practice can improve your mood and sleep quality, reduce stress and increase your strength, flexibility and balance. It is possible to learn tai chi at home with online tuition, but it's often best to learn how to perform the movements correctly by joining a class. Learning with others is also a great way to make new friends and enjoy the mood-enhancing effects of belonging to a social network.

Think about therapy

If your low mood persists, your medical practitioner may refer you to a counsellor or a psychotherapist. While some argue that overanalyzing your life can make depression worse, many people find it helpful to talk things over with someone they can trust. Often, it's a huge relief to realize that what you're going through is normal. Also, some therapists encourage you to think more positively, which has been shown to help lift low mood. Counselling is usually a short-term treatment (less than six months) for people who have a specific problem to deal with or who are finding it hard to cope with a stressful event, such as divorce or bereavement. A counsellor doesn't normally offer advice, but instead helps you to better understand yourself, your feelings and behaviour. They will also work on your self-esteem and ability to take control of your own life.

Clue up on counselling

There are two main types of counselling: directive, where the counsellor determines the structure of sessions; and non-directive, where you decide what is discussed. Directive forms of counselling include Cognitive Behavioural Therapy (CBT) and Gestalt counselling.

Non-directive includes psychodynamic and person-centred counselling. The next couple of pages will give you more insight into each approach to help you choose the best type for your particular issue.

Directive counselling

Cognitive Behavioural Therapy (CBT) and Gestalt counselling are types of directive counselling. In CBT counselling you are encouraged to recognize the negative thought patterns that may be involved in your low mood or anxiety and replace them with more realistic and positive ones. The counsellor may ask you to keep a diary of your thoughts and feelings. Gestalt counselling focuses on your thoughts, feelings and activity patterns, and promotes self-awareness. You learn how to improve your self-awareness by assessing your behaviour and body language, as well as expressing any suppressed feelings. Sessions can include acting out difficult scenarios and conversations, in addition to remembering dreams.

Non-directive counselling

Psychodynamic counselling is a form of non-directive counselling based on the idea that previous events in your life affect what you feel and experience now. Your counsellor will ask you about your past, focusing on areas such as your childhood, family and relationships. They will help you to understand how these are impacting your emotions and actions now, which can help you to break free from your past if it's holding you back.

Person-centred counselling is based on the idea that you are the best person to solve your own problems. The counsellor offers empathy, positive feedback, honesty and openness to encourage you to share and understand the emotions that have led to your depression. This develops your self-awareness and confidence, and empowers you to identify and resolve the issues that underpin your low mood.

Psychotherapy

Psychotherapy may be suggested if you have long-term depression that doesn't seem to be associated with a specific event in your life, but which could be down to more deep-rooted emotional issues. Nowadays there is less of a distinction between counselling and psychotherapy, but generally counsellors undertake shorter training than psychotherapists. As with counselling, psychotherapy is based on certain theories, such as Cognitive Behavioural Therapy (CBT) or psychodynamic therapy. Psychotherapy usually goes on for longer than counselling, often for several months or more. It's also more in-depth and tends to concentrate on deeply ingrained ways of thinking that might have developed during your childhood.

Antidepressants – it's your decision

Depression is usually caused by a combination of factors and it's only by addressing these that you will get better. The best advice is to first follow the tips in this book – manage your stress levels, tackle negative thought patterns, eat well and take regular exercise. But if these lifestyle changes don't help and your depression is severely affecting your ability to cope with daily life, or making you suicidal, speak to your medical practitioner. They may be happy to refer you for CBT, but they may also want to prescribe an antidepressant. Whether or not you decide to take one is ultimately up to you. Antidepressants exert a powerful effect on the brain to change the levels of neurotransmitters, which may be necessary if you have moderate to severe depression. However, your decision to take them must be weighed up against their potential side effects.

Learn about antidepressants

Antidepressants are medications used to relieve moderate to severe depression by increasing the levels of neurotransmitters – the chemicals that transmit messages from nerve cells in the brain. The three most involved in depression are serotonin, the happy hormone, and get-up-and-go hormones, adrenaline and noradrenaline. The use of antidepressants stems from the theory that depression is caused by low levels of one or more of these neurotransmitters. Although this may be an oversimplified view, boosting neurotransmitters can improve low mood, especially alongside a talking therapy like Cognitive Behavioural Therapy (CBT). It may take a few weeks to notice any improvement and, like most medications, antidepressants can cause side effects. Most are mild and usually settle down in time. Common side effects include a dry mouth, drowsiness, dizziness, constipation and weight gain. Be aware that antidepressants can interact with other medicines including ibuprofen, aspirin and triptans – a treatment for migraines.

SSRIs explained

Selective serotonin reuptake inhibitors (SSRIs) raise levels of serotonin in the brain by stopping it being reabsorbed into the nerve cells. They are called selective because they mainly affect serotonin levels. They include citalopram (Cipramil, Celexa), escitalopram (Cipralex, Lexapro), fluoxetine (Prozac), fluvoxamine (Faverin, Luvox), paroxetine (Seroxat, Paxil) and sertraline (Lustral, Zoloft). Although SSRIs are less likely to cause side effects than older antidepressants, they may still cause some unwanted effects. SSRIs aren't recommended if you have bipolar disorder, poorly controlled epilepsy, severe liver impairment or an abnormal heart rhythm.

SNRIs explained

Selective serotonin and noradrenaline reuptake inhibitors (SNRIs) increase levels of mood-boosting serotonin and energizing noradrenaline in the brain. They include venlafaxine (Effexor) and duloxetine (Cymbalta and Irenka). You shouldn't take an SNRI if you have untreated high blood pressure (hypertension), an arrhythmia (irregular heartbeat) or have liver or kidney disease.

TCAs explained

Tricyclics (TCAs) also raise levels of noradrenaline and serotonin in the brain. Tricyclic antidepressants include amitriptyline (Elavil), dosulepin (formerly dothiepin), imipramine (Tofranil), lofepramine, nortriptyline and clomipramine. These are an older class of antidepressant that are used less often nowadays, although they can work well for severe depression that hasn't responded to other treatments. They can improve sleep, so are useful for people who also suffer from insomnia. They are also used to treat chronic pain and prevent migraines. You shouldn't be prescribed a tricyclic if you are recovering from a heart attack or if you have bipolar, kidney or liver disease, diabetes or a heart rhythm disorder.

SARIs explained

Serotonin antagonists and reuptake inhibitors (SARIs) also boost levels of the good mood hormone, serotonin. These are not usually the first choice of antidepressant, but they may be prescribed if other antidepressants haven't helped or have caused intolerable side-effects. Examples of this kind of medication include trazodone (Molipaxin) and nefazodone (Serzone). SARIs shouldn't be taken if you have liver problems.

MAOIs explained

Monoamine oxidase inhibitors (MAOIs) are an older group of drugs that increase levels of noradrenaline (also known as norepinephrine) and serotonin in the brain. They include phenelzine, isocarboxazid, tranylcypromine and moclobemide. A major problem with them is they can interact with certain other drugs and tyramine-rich foods and drinks such as mature cheeses, processed meats (salami, pepperoni), pickled herrings, broad beans, fermented soya bean extract, yeast extracts (Bovril, Oxo, Marmite) and most alcoholic and low-alcohol drinks, to cause severe high blood pressure and other conditions. MAOIs shouldn't be taken during pregnancy or alongside other antidepressants.

NASSAs explained

Noradrenaline and specific serotonergic antidepressants (NASSAs) also raise levels of serotonin and noradrenaline and can be effective for some people who can't tolerate SSRIs. However, they may cause more drowsiness than other antidepressants when you first start taking them. Examples of this type of medication include Mirtazapine (Remeron, Avanza, Zispin), Trazodone and Mianserin (Tolvon). They shouldn't be prescribed if you have an irregular heartbeat or high blood pressure.

Referral to a mental health specialist

If your depression isn't relieved with the lifestyle changes, talking treatments or antidepressants discussed in this book or is especially severe, your medical practitioner may refer you to a mental health specialist, such as a psychiatrist or a clinical psychologist who will be able to reassess your condition and devise a more in-depth treatment plan for you. A psychiatrist will look at both your physical and mental health before making a diagnosis and prescribing medication. They may also refer you to a psychologist or a particular type of therapist.

Get to the point

If you would prefer to try alternative treatments you might want to consider acupuncture, as there is evidence it can help to ease depression. Traditional acupuncture is a branch of Chinese medicine dating back 2,000 years. It involves inserting ultra-fine needles into certain points on the body to restore the flow of qi (natural energy) and invoke a healing response. It's thought to treat depression by boosting levels of feel-good endorphins and happy hormones, serotonin and dopamine, while encouraging relaxation and reducing stress levels. If you decide to try this treatment, choose an acupuncturist who is a healthcare professional or a registered member of a recognized acupuncture organization.

Scents of calm

Essential oils come from the petals, leaves, stalk, roots, seeds, nuts or the bark of plants, and are another way we can improve our well-being through engaging with nature. Aromatherapy is based on the principle that when scents from essential oils are inhaled, they affect the hypothalamus. This part of the brain controls the glands and hormones, so it's thought that these oils can enhance mood to reduce stress and anxiety levels. When used in massage, baths and compresses, the oils are absorbed through the skin into the bloodstream and carried to the organs and glands, which benefit from their healing properties. Several oils are believed to ease depression so choose the ones that could help your particular symptoms. Citrussy oils like bergamot and grapefruit have uplifting and energizing properties, while fragrant rose oil is both comforting and uplifting – it is especially recommended for grief and loss. Earthy-scented lavender is a great stress reliever and is hard to beat when it comes to easing tension, relaxing tight muscles and promoting sound sleep. Try it in a massage before bed or sprinkle a few drops on your pillow at night. Sweet-smelling neroli is also soothing at bedtime and helps relieve anxiety. Try adding a few drops to your shower gel or add a little to a warm bath.

Make time for a massage

Massage is a tried and tested way to alleviate stress and anxiety. To make your own massage oil simply add an essential oil of your choice to a good quality carrier oil. You can use vegetable or sunflower oil, as well as almond, sesame seed or grapeseed oils. Add the essential oil at a ratio of six drops to a tablespoon of carrier oil.

Never apply aromatherapy oils to broken skin. Buy the best quality oils you can afford because cheaper oils may not be as pure as more costly ones. If you have sensitive skin, do a patch test before trying an essential oil you haven't used before. Rub a few drops of diluted oil inside your wrist or elbow. If there's no reaction within 24 hours it should be safe to use.

The sound of music

Music can affect our emotions and motivate or comfort us, as well as give us pleasure. Your musical tastes can also be strongly tied to your sense of who you are. Listening to music can be a great way to regulate your emotions, especially if you create playlists to suit your different moods. When you feel anxious or are having trouble sleeping, choose music you find calming – classical tunes might fit the bill. When you need to lighten your mood, select songs with upbeat tunes and happy, light-hearted lyrics. If you're lacking in energy, pick music with a fast tempo to uplift you. Sometimes you might just want to listen to sad songs that reflect how you're feeling. This is also fine, as long as they don't exacerbate your low mood.

Feel happier – fast!

Sometimes when your mood is low you might need a quick boost to get you back on track. Any one of these tips could help:

- Smile. Smiling releases endorphins, dopamine and serotonin, which quickly boosts your mood.

- Sit and stand up straight. Holding your spine straight allows happy hormones like serotonin and endorphins to flow more easily.

- Look up. Looking upward lifts your mood by encouraging your brain to produce more calming alpha waves.

- Take a cold shower. Turning the setting to cold for the last minute of your daily shower encourages your body to release the mood-enhancing hormone, noradrenaline.

- Get crafty. Sewing and knitting are forms of mindfulness that can take your attention away from your problems and alleviate depression.

Conclusion

Hopefully this book has helped you identify the underlying reasons for your depression, as well as the steps you can take to address them and get on the road to recovery. Understanding which foods and physical activities can boost your outlook will enable you to make better lifestyle choices for improved mental wellbeing, while learning about the types of antidepressants you may be offered when you're at your lowest ebb means you can make an informed decision on whether to take them or not. Adopting a more positive outlook will help you to become more resilient in the face of adversity. Following the simple suggestions to dial down your stress levels will lead to a healthier mindset. Above all, remember that while depression cannot always be cured, it is possible to alleviate your symptoms to enjoy a happier, healthier and more fulfilled life.

About the Author

Wendy Green is a health project co-ordinator and health promoter, and the author of a wide range of health books in the Vie list, including *Anxiety: A Self-Help Guide to Feeling Better*, *100 Tips to Help You Through the Menopause*, *The Happy Gut Guide* and *The New Parents' Survival Guide: The First Three Months*.

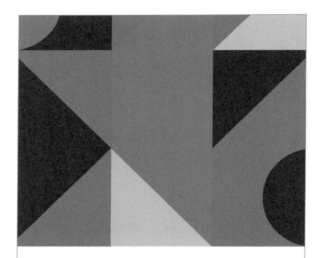

How to Understand and Deal With

Anxiety

RASHA BARRAGE

HOW TO UNDERSTAND AND DEAL WITH ANXIETY

Rasha Barrage

£6.99
ISBN: 978-1-80007-425-5
Paperback

Feeling overwhelmed?
This little book is here to help.

By the end of this friendly, accessible guide, you will:

- Understand the science behind anxiety, how it manifests, what causes it, and how to identify symptoms and triggers

- Be armed with physical and practical steps you can take to alleviate anxiety, from breathing exercises and healthy lifestyle choices to problem-solving techniques and coping mechanisms

- Have a host of holistic remedies up your sleeve for when anxiety strikes, such as mindfulness, visualization and breathwork

- Know about the medical treatments and therapies available, and know how and when to seek professional help or support

If you're interested in finding out more about our books, find us on Facebook at **Summersdale Publishers**, on Twitter at **@Summersdale** and on Instagram at **@summersdalebooks** and get in touch.

Thanks very much for buying this Summersdale book.

www.summersdale.com